What is the Keto Diet?

HOW TO AVOID MISTAKES AND GET RESULTS (BEGINNER'S GUIDE)

TINA LEE

WHAT IS THE KETO DIET?

CONTENTS

Part 1.
Something about Keto

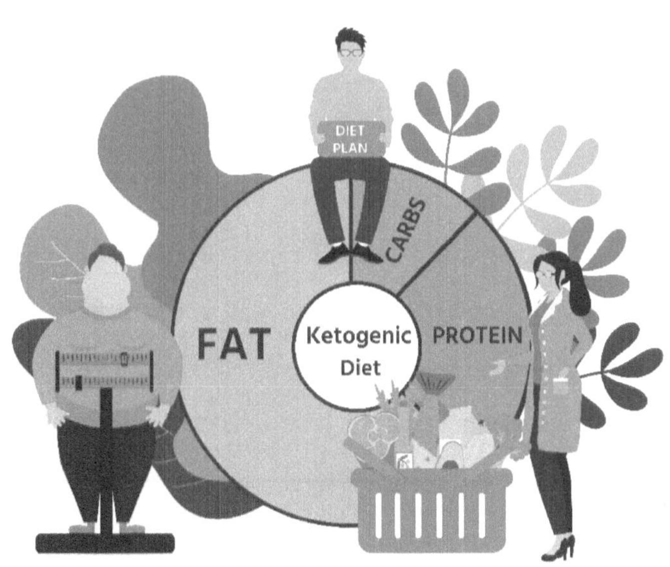

Keto diet - where did it come from and how does it work?

Keto, Ketogenic, has become viral throughout the web and especially on social media platforms. But this ancient diet has been around for quite a long time; we just didn't know enough about it.

This is not a novelty.

The classic ketogenic diet has formed in the 1920s, when doctors applied the keto approach to patients who suffered from epilepsy, to control the seizures. This method also worked with patients who suffered from other diseases such as diabetes and several types of nervous disorders. The low carb high-fat diet was used as a therapy for various types of neurological disorders such as Alzheimer, sleep disorders, Parkinson's disease, brain cancer and other similar disorders.

Keto diet follows the role of fasting for treating diseases. This method has been around for ages particularly during Ancient Greece. Hippocrates wrote that hunger contributes to the reduction of epilepsy attacks. However, no patient could go hungry forever, so doctors tried to make an adequate menu. Despite such an ancient origin of the diet the first research that was conducted was in France in 1911 when the diet was found to improve patients' mental problems. Already in 1924, after two years of research, the ketogenic diet was officially recorded and began to be used to treat epilepsy.

It was found that ketone bodies, which are released in the human body in the process of fasting, have a positive effect on the reduction of epilepsy attacks. It is surprising that if a patient drew energy from food rich in fats, containing moderate amounts of proteins in the complete absence of carbohydrates, then the process of ketone body production did not stop. The therapeutic effect accumulated, intensified and at the same time the patient did not starve!

Such treatment is applied not only to adults but also to children. Children who suffered from seizures were placed in a keto diet program where a doctor and a nutritionist prepare a strict meal plan for them to follow. The meal plan consists of almost 90% calories that come from fats with no carbohydrates and restricted protein amounts. The treatment course can vary from one child to another. Some only need to follow the keto diet for 3 months while other patients who still encounter seizures might need to continue with the keto diet for up to 2 years. Studies have shown that most patients who followed the keto diet have had decreased seizures or stopped completely.

The success of the keto diet was overwhelming and did not stop even in the late 30s when in 1938 the first antiepileptic drugs were created.

And yet, with the development of pharmacology in subsequent years, interest in the diet has decreased markedly. Anti-convulsive drugs allowed patients not to adhere to strict food restrictions. The diet was called an obsolete method, and for some time it was dismissed. It took time to realize that the new therapies didn't work with almost 30% of patients with epilepsy and new pharmaceuticals had many side effects that were especially dangerous for children. Already in the early 70s, a light Medium-Chain Triglyceride oil diet was created, which was included in the treatment program to control the disease.

Another problem was that the keto-diet was considered as an aid only to patients with epilepsy and the possibility of applying it to other diagnoses was not considered.

Some revival of the diet occurred in the 60s when Atkins proposed a similar nutritional system in order to control weight. Unfortunately, the Atkins diet very quickly became similar to a commercial idea, and after a while interest in it was lost. Besides Keto diet was also highlighted in the 1990's when it was exposed on media through Jim Abraham's movie, Do Not Harm. In the movie a young boy is diagnosed with epilepsy and his parents agree to force him to undertake excruciating treatments that only worsened his condition. Later on, his doctor learns about the Keto diet and how it was used before to treat patients with epilepsy. He learnt that patients who followed the diet no longer suffered from additional seizures. The film is based on real events and attracted drew attention to how Keto diet can be used not just for a healthier lifestyle but for also treating medical diseases.

On our time, the use of ketosis is not limited to epilepsy. The practice has shown that low-carbohydrate nutrition can make life easier for those who suffer from diseases such as epilepsy, obesity, cancer, diabetes, CNS diseases, neurodegenerative diseases, autoimmune diseases. It is also useful for any inflammations and at the same time, patients do not need to endure exhausting starvation.

Keto diet is still effective

In world full of all types and kinds of diets, what makes Keto successful? How does it really work?

The magic behind the success of the keto diet is by changing the mechanism of energy-producing in our bodies. Many have heard about the benefits of fasting for physical health. In terms of metabolism, fasting and keto diet are very similar. Our bodies are used to burning carbohydrates for energy so minimizing carbohydrates intake will cause your body to break down stored fat to use as energy. Keto diet like fasting forced our bodies to enter a state known at Ketosis when the body starts producing Ketones. This is a physiological state that converts stored fat into the energy source. The essential difference between keto diets and fasting is that the person continues to eat and the effect of fasting does not stop! This is the foundation of the entire diet, and this is what you need to remember when making an individual nutrition plan.

With not enough glucose in the system, your body will find an alternative energy source. Therefore it starts breaking down fat stores to obtain the glucose from triglycerides.

The keto diet consists of around 5% carbs, 20% protein and 75% healthy fats. Following this diet will help with weight loss because all the consumed fat will keep you full throughout the day and away from "snacking" on restricted food. This is also an important principle. It is very difficult for many to recognize the fact that fats can be beneficial.

Many of us have already developed a dependence on carbohydrates because they predominate in the diet of modern man. Refusal of them leads to a serious restructuring of the body, which is accompanied by weakness, irritability and other unpleasant symptoms.

Perhaps you are already familiar with the principles of Keto diets and even started to follow it. It may be very important for you to reduce the consumption of carbohydrates because of your health, but you always stop. I am not a doctor. But many times I had to communicate with my clients who, for one reason or another, tried to stick to ketogenic nutrition. They needed support and I felt that I had to sort out this issue to help them. I had to read a lot, communicate with doctors and nutritionists. It is not in my competence to recommend you a keto diet or discourage you from it. Your doctor should do this. But if you decide to follow it, then I want to help you not to make the most frequent mistakes that are typical of beginners.

A small dictionary so as not to get confused

In this book you will come across these terms repetitively

Ketosis

Is a metabolic state that occurs when the ketone bodies levels are raised in the body tissues. This happens when glucose levels are low so the body uses stored fat as an alternative energy source.

Ketone Bodies

Water-soluble molecules produced by the liver during ketosis state

Ketoacidosis

When the body enters ketosis phase and starts producing ketone bodies to use as an energy source; the level of produced ketone bodies can become too high. In this case, the blood becomes more acidic and this condition is known as ketoacidosis. It is a life-threatening condition with symptoms such as nausea, abdominal pain and rapid breathing. It is also known as diabetic ketoacidosis.

Low Carb Diet

A diet that restricts the amount of carbohydrates intake and focuses on higher levels of protein and healthy fat intake. There are different types of low-carb diets, each one with its own restrictions and benefits.

Triglycerides

Triglycerides are the main energy reserve of a person, it is these substances that accumulate in the cells of adipose tissue. The body receives triglycerides with food and also synthesizes them from other nutrient substances, such as carbohydrates. When the body experiences energy hunger, it breaks down triglycerides with the release of water, glycerin, and energy.

So maybe all we need is a keto?

Following any diet, you must know that nothing is perfect and there are side effects and disadvantages to any program. The bottom line is that we cannot live without food. After all, from it, we get the building material for our organs and all body systems. Most often under the diet means some restrictions on food. This means that some substances entered into our body, and some do not. Changes in nutrition will invariably lead to changes in the work of our body. What will be the result? Healthy or vice versa, will harm our health. Therefore before following a certain diet you must be well aware of it, read enough about it and most importantly checked with a doctor or nutritionist first. Not everyone is fit to follow a specific diet having to adjust the diet to meet their special needs.

Keto diet can be very useful for diseases such as cardiovascular disease, metabolic syndromes, diabetes, and nervous disorders. It was also found to help control cholesterol levels and promoting weight loss.

There is ongoing research to confirm if the keto diet helps with other diseases such as Parkinson's, Alzheimer, and some cancer types.

The undoubted advantage of keto-diet is that it does not offer to use products created by modern industry, deprived of natural ingredients necessary for health. This brings us back to the natural food that has been around for thousands of years, leading to many positive results. Let's talk about them in more detail.

Undeniable Benefits

One of the most known benefits of the keto diet is weight loss and it's probably what most people who follow the diet are aiming for. Although this is not the reason why the Keto diet appeared, it is a pretty welcome addition for those who decide to stick to a Keto diet due to serious health problems.

Keto diet improves insulin resistance by lowering blood sugar levels. Modern industry has made sugar quickly available. Refined foods are really evil, they are devoid of ballast substances that make their absorption slow and natural for our body. Think about what kind of work our body needs to sell to get a couple of teaspoons of sugar from the foods we ate. For example, an apple. Fresh apple contains a whole complex of vitamins and minerals. 85% of it consists of water, the remaining 15% are carbohydrates and proteins, fiber, ash, and starch. The amount of sugar is quite low: in a fresh apple of the average size it is about 20 grams, and if it is a green apple variety, then even less. So, in one apple about 2-3 teaspoons of sugar. But for them to enter the bloodstream, the body needs to work hard. So this portion of sugar will enter the human blood gradually over the course of several hours, literally bit by bit. But refined sugar will enter our bloodstream instantly as soon as we taste it in our tongue!

High blood sugar leads to many other health problems, and hair and skin often suffer in the first place.

Research has proven that the keto diet might help in preventing cancer. One research has suggested cancer patients can follow a keto diet while taking chemotherapy.

Other research has shown that the keto diet can help prevent diseases such as Parkinson's, Alzheimer and sleep disorder conditions.

Another interesting benefit of the keto diet is for women who suffer from Polycystic ovarian syndrome (PCOS), Patients with PCOS cannot follow a high carbohydrates diet as it can be very harmful to them. There hasn't been much research conducted in this field but one research has tested a group of women with PCOS for 24 weeks. The results were improved hormone balanced, fasting insulin and faster weight loss.

The low carb keto diet aids weight loss and the good news is that the larger proportion of fat loss comes from the abdominal area and this is most common for overweight men. Therefore following the keto diet can be really effective in reducing fat in those tricky areas, because the abdominal area is where most of the organs are found: liver, stomach and the heart. The lower the fat stored around these organs and lower the risk for heart disease in the future.

But fat is not only stored under the skin and around organs, but it can also be found in the bloodstream, known as triglycerides. Keto diet helps to lower Triglycerides levels in the bloodstream. This is linked to heart diseases as high levels of triglycerides are strong factors for heart disease risk.

Another risk associated with diabetes is metabolic syndrome.

Symptoms of this condition include raised blood pressure and fasting blood sugar levels, low good cholesterol levels, and high triglycerides. The good news is following a low carb diet has been shown to be quite effective in treating these symptoms.

You will probably notice that many benefits of the keto diet are related to blood pressure and heart diseases. That's correct by following a low carb diet you are reducing of heart disease as the bad cholesterol particles in your bloodstream are reduced.

For a modern person, weight loss and lowering cholesterol seem incredible when eating, in which you need to eat a considerable amount of fat. After all, for several decades we considered fats to be our worst enemy. But as the practice has shown, the exclusion of fat from daily food has not made us healthier. Fats of plant and animal origin are an integral part of a healthy immune, hormonal and respiratory systems.

In principle, a balanced keto diet is a natural way of eating for a person who lived a couple of hundred years ago when there were no modern, refined, fat-free and "improved" foods.

Caution: Keto diet!

Just like everything else in life, there are always disadvantages and risks and keto diet is no exception.

Even though there are health benefits and successful treatment for diseases and nervous disorders, a keto diet can be very dangerous if not properly observed.

Please keep in mind that not all body types are the same. We don't all function the same way as others. It is very important to understand how your body works to be able to meet its needs.

1. **Nutrient deficiency.** One of the biggest drawbacks of the keto diet is a nutrient deficiency, as the diet limits carbohydrate intake, which means that you are cut off from many fruits, vegetables, and cereals. This will cause nutrition deficiency which might also lead to conditions such as kidney stones, gallbladder issues, and bone fracture.

2. **'Keto flu'.** Once you start the keto diet you will experience a common condition known as 'keto flu'. It's the ugly part of the process of transforming your body into ketosis mode. Symptoms include nausea, vomiting, dizziness, weakness, irritability, headaches, and constipation. This happens when your body starts producing ketones and tries to get rid of it through urine. Alongside experiencing these symptoms you are also prompt to have sugar cravings and difficult concentration.

3. **Losing electrolytes.** As the keto flu takes place your body is losing all its electrolytes by frequent urination, you are on the risk of losing too much. Such essential electrolytes include potassium, sodium, and magnesium. Lack of these minerals can cause kidney failure.

4. **Dehydration.** Another dangerous hazard is that your body will face dehydration by the frequent urination and this can lead to irregular heartbeats and thus resulting in serious deadly heart issues.

5. **Frequent change in eating style.** Following such a strict diet like keto is that most people have a hard time sticking to it and end up giving up. Others might give up for a while and jump into trying a different diet or resume with keto again. This diet switching can be very dangerous and cause weight fluctuations and increases mortality risks. Your body takes time to adjust to a certain diet and changing it every now and then will confuse your body system and you'll be facing major health issues.

6. **Bad breath**. But not all hazards are deadly there are also minor disadvantages when following keto diet such as: bad breath - this is inevitable. As your body produces ketones it also tries to get rid of it. It does that through exhalation and ketones smell like acetone-literally. This strong-foul smell can be extremely uncomfortable during the ketosis phase and usually, it lingers for a long time. You are advised to drink a lot of fluids to wash it down but it won't go away, Other solutions will include sugar-free gum to cover up the scent.

7. **Loss of muscle tissue**. Although keto guarantees weight loss and reduces the risk of certain types of diseases, prolonged exposure to keto can lead to loss of muscle tissue. Protein is essential for muscles we all know that but muscles also need carbohydrates for muscle formation. When your body is in ketosis mode for a long time, it will rely on just fats for energy. This leaving you consuming fewer calories because the fat will satisfy your hunger for long hours. This can be helpful for

weight loss but over time your body is lacking the necessary calories it needs so it starts to lose muscle tissue, which results in muscle loss from the heart as well leading to damage to tissue cells.

* * *

However, most of these effects can be successfully avoided. Let's look at the most common mistakes that newcomers to the keto diet make and see how to avoid them.